© Aladdin Books Ltd 1987

Designed and produced by
Aladdin Books Ltd
70 Old Compton Street
London W1

*First published in the
United States in 1987 by*
Franklin Watts
387 Park Avenue South
New York NY 10016

ISBN 0-531 10435 4

Library of Congress Catalog
Card Number: 87-50600

Printed in Belgium

*The publishers wish to thank those involved in
producing this book, especially Dr John Fry,
medical doctor and author*

Design	David West Children's Book Design
Editor	Steve Parker
Researcher	Cecilia Weston-Baker
Illustrator	Peter Harper

Contents

UNDERSTANDING DRUGS

COCAINE AND CRACK

Julian Chomet

FRANKLIN WATTS
New York · London · Toronto · Sydney

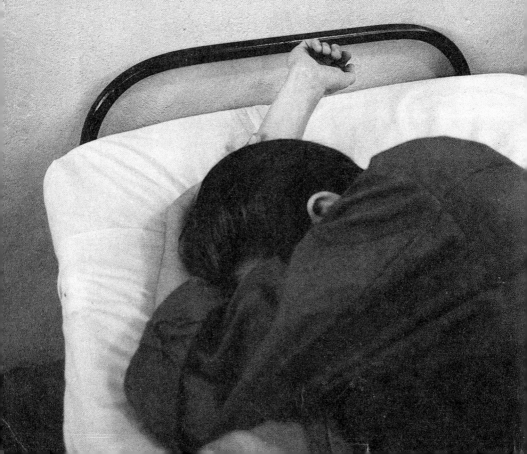

INTRODUCTION

In the 1960s and 1970s the drug cocaine became famous as the "plaything" of the rich and famous. Movie stars and musicians would "tell all" to the newspapers in sensational stories about their wild parties and their cocaine addiction. Somehow the drug became linked with a glamorous and successful lifestyle. What didn't come through in the newspaper stories were the terrible effects the drug could have on people's lives.

At that time, cocaine was so expensive that it was out of reach of most people. However the last few years have seen a flood of cheap cocaine into North America and Europe. It is now a problem right across all levels of society, from top actors and sports stars down to the ordinary people in the street.

The cost to the victims of cocaine is not only in money. Their health worsens. They may take to crime to pay for their drug habit. In the end, the ultimate payment can be death.

In the last few years, a new form of cocaine has begun to take hold. This is crack, which has been described as "the most dangerous and the most addictive drug" ever available to the public. Since it first appeared on the streets in 1984, crack has become widespread throughout the

The dangers of drugs: solving nothing, simply adding problems.

United States and has begun to appear in other countries.

One reason for the cocaine and crack explosion is the cost, which is now so low that almost anyone can afford to buy the drugs. Also the myth is still around that cocaine is a harmless drug which can be controlled by the user, without leading to addiction. But graveyards, hospitals and drug treatment centers are full of people who believed this to be true.

It may be tempting to try cocaine, or even crack, to see what all the fuss is about. This book tells you about some of the consequences of taking cocaine and crack. It tells you what can happen to your mind and body and how easily you can become addicted.

Other names for cocaine

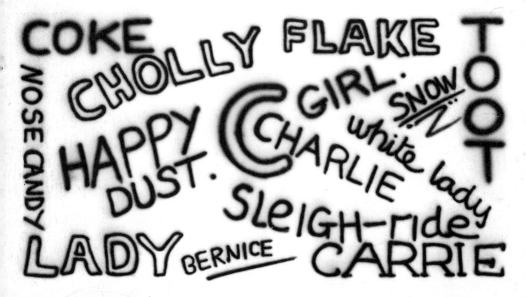

WHY TAKE COCAINE AND CRACK?

❝ If you want to get down, down on the ground – cocaine. ❞

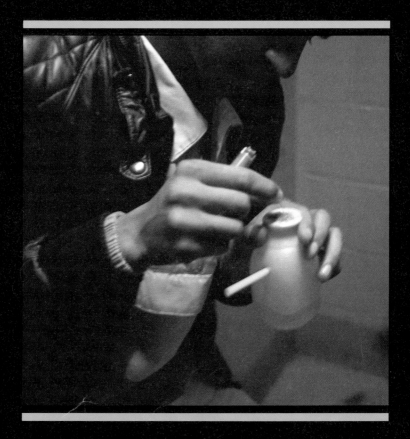

> **If you want to get down, down on the ground – cocaine.** 99

You are at a party. Someone has some drugs. Everyone seems to be having a wild time and someone offers you some white powder to sniff or a strange cigarette to smoke. They say it will make you feel great. "Go on, everyone is taking it. Enjoy yourself. Don't be boring." What do you do?

Social pressure

This social pressure, being urged by others, is one of the main reasons why people try drugs like cocaine and crack. Say no, and you might feel you're being boring. But say yes and you're agreeing to experiment with something un-known. What effects will it have on you? It's no good looking at its effects on others, since everyone reacts differently. You could be the one whose "yes" will lead to a lifetime of addiction and misery.

Taking cocaine or crack might seem daring or exciting, but people whose lives have been ruined probably wished they had known more at the time.

> **It was a party and everyone was up. It was the worst day of my life.** 99

Drugs are sold and used openly, even in "amusement" arcades.

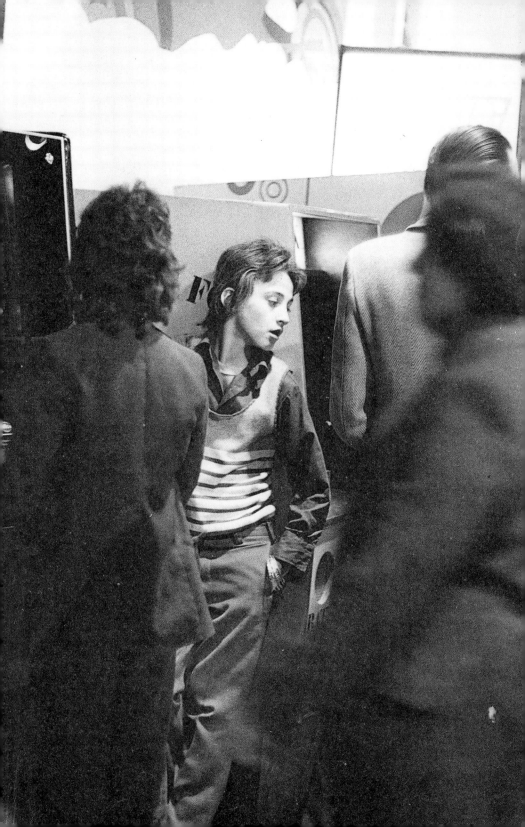

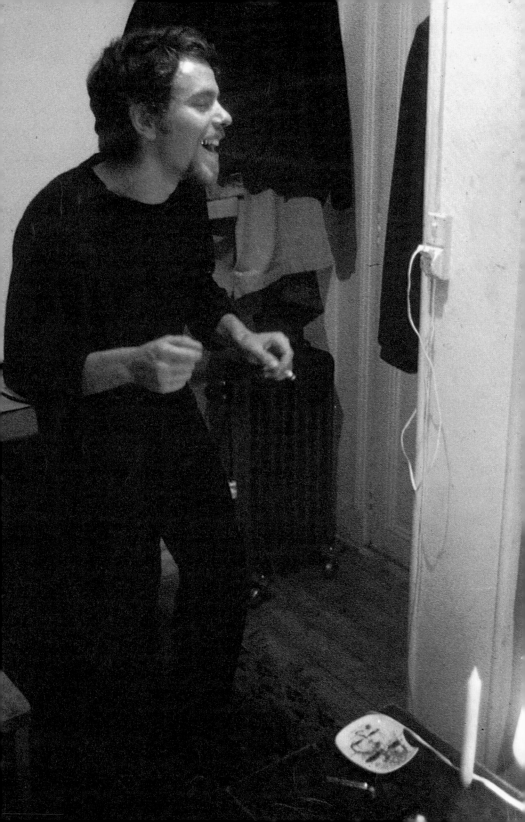

Cost and availability

Because cocaine and crack have become relatively cheap, there is plenty around. Cocaine is no longer a drug of the rich. Kids on the streets of every major city – and now in the small towns and country areas too – are being arrested for possessing drugs like cocaine and crack. So it's becoming more likely that you may be offered some.

I take it because . . .

There are many reasons why people agree to take drugs like cocaine, aside from pressure from their friends or elders. There's the excitement of doing something that's illegal and a protest against authority. There's also the excuse that drug-taking is fashionable, it's "the thing to do." All the cool people do it. Of course, in real life this isn't true. Very few truly successful and stylish people take drugs, and usually we get to hear about them because of the way cocaine or crack messes them up.

Another excuse is that "everything is so boring." Life seems dull and tedious, full of hassles. Drugs offer excitement. In the end, though, drugs like cocaine and crack don't solve anything. They simply make things worse.

Why should some people turn to cocaine and crack in particular, and not to other drugs? Probably they have heard about the feelings they give, of the pleasure and energy and exhilaration. Is this really true?

High on drugs, but how bumpy will the "crash" landing be?

What does cocaine do?

Cocaine is usually taken by "snorting" (sniffing it up the nose). It passes through the thin lining inside the nose into the blood beneath and is then carried to the brain. The feelings it causes are due to its effects on the brain.

When someone takes cocaine, they feel a short period of exhilaration, often called a buzz, high, rush or trip. This starts after about three minutes and fades over the next hour. The user has a sense of physical and mental power, of feeling extra-alert and extremely happy (euphoria). He forgets about hunger, and any tiredness seems to be replaced by a new-found energy.

The "energy" effect is why many users take cocaine, to try and get them through their work when they need plenty of stamina, concentration and imagination.

What does crack do?

Crack is usually heated in some way, and the vapors it gives off are breathed into the lungs, like cigarette smoke. Its effects are similar to cocaine, except that the feelings come on much faster, often within seconds. This is because the lining of the lungs is very thin and has a great surface area. So the drug is absorbed very quickly into the blood and travels to the brain in one powerful punch, whereas snorting cocaine has a more drawn-out effect.

The initial high of crack is like the high of cocaine, but stronger, more powerful and intense. It lasts only around five minutes, and the effects wear off after about 15 to 20 minutes.

> **♥♥ I was high, man, was I high. It was like a bird, way up above the earth, feeling so good. 🙌**

Unfortunately there is a price to pay for these moments of "pleasure." For these aren't the only effects of cocaine and crack. There are plenty of problems, too.

The problems

One problem with any street drug is that users never really know how safe it is. Sometimes pure drugs are mixed with other substances. This can easily lead to high doses being snorted. The results may be very unpleasant, such as being confused and suspicious about everyone and everything (paranoia). High doses may also make the skin extremely sensitive, giving the feeling of bugs crawling all over the body. The pupils get bigger and the heartbeat speeds up.

Cocaine has many and widespread bad effects on the body.

*worry and anxiety

*hallucinations

*widened (dilated) pupils of the eyes

*increased heartbeat rate

*damaged heart muscle

*inability to sleep

*weight loss

*confusion and suspicion (paranoia)

The higher and longer the cocaine "trip" lasts, the bumpier the landing is on coming down – the "crash." Repeated use can lead to weight loss, worry and anxiety, and an inability to sleep (insomnia). The person may experience frightening hallucinations of seeing or hearing terrible things, and this could lead to violent behavior.

Damage from regular use

There are many damaging effects to health from regular cocaine use. Frequent snorting can cause nosebleeds and painful, sore ulcers on the nasal septum, the soft flap inside the nose that separates the two nostrils.

More seriously, the heartbeat and breathing lose their steady rhythm. The user pants quickly and then suddenly takes large gulps of air. The end result may be a heart attack and possibly death.

There is also evidence that cocaine damages the muscle of the heart, which may explain why otherwise healthy people suddenly die of an overdose. Like lung cancer and smoking cigarettes, this type of danger from cocaine is long-term. Taking cocaine now may make a heart attack more likely in the future. There is also recent evidence that cocaine use may upset the delicate chemical balance of the brain and possibly speed up the ageing process.

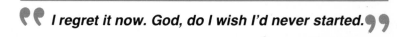

 ❝ *I regret it now. God, do I wish I'd never started.* ❞

WHERE DO THEY COME FROM?

"Cocaine can make the most dismal melancholic cheerful."

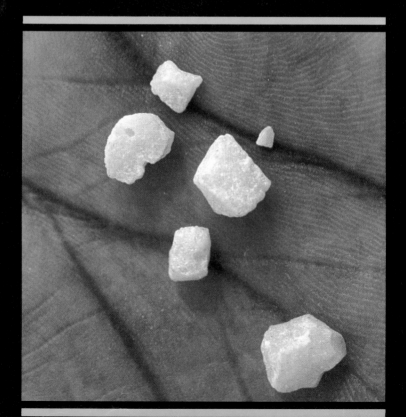

There is nothing new about cocaine. It has been around for more than a hundred years. Late in the last century it was used widely by doctors, who prescribed it for their patients for a variety of illnesses, particularly depression. It was a drug that was used as a mild stimulant.

❝ *Cocaine can make the most dismal melancholic cheerful." A doctor speaking in the last century.* **❞**

Cocaine the "wonder drug"

In a pure but weak form, cocaine was available from drug stores all over the United States. There were cocaine cigarettes, and cocaine inhalants were manufactured by the medical companies. The drug was even found in Coca-

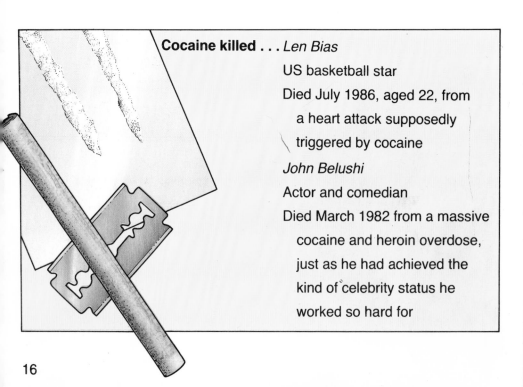

Cocaine killed . . . *Len Bias*
US basketball star
Died July 1986, aged 22, from
 a heart attack supposedly
 triggered by cocaine
John Belushi
Actor and comedian
Died March 1982 from a massive
 cocaine and heroin overdose,
 just as he had achieved the
 kind of celebrity status he
 worked so hard for

Cola, although once its dangers were noticed it was removed, in 1903.

The first epidemic of cocaine use began in about 1885. Sigmund Freud, the famous "father of psychoanalysis," made the drug popular in Europe by pointing to its praise in US medical journals. European doctors began to recommend cocaine for various illnesses, especially depression, just as their American counterparts did.

But soon the unpleasant effects of the drug were noticed. By 1891 it was clear that cocaine was dangerous and it quickly disappeared from medicine. The US authorities effectively banned cocaine under the Harrison Narcotic Act of 1914. It was similarly banned in Britain in 1916.

What does cocaine look like?

Cocaine is a whitish powder, usually made of small shiny crystals. It has no smell but does have a bitter flavor. When it comes into contact with the tongue, lips or nose it causes a gradual numbness.

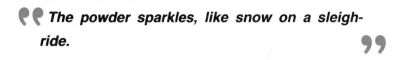

❝❝ *The powder sparkles, like snow on a sleigh-ride.* **❞❞**

Cocaine powder is made from the leaves of the South American coca plant, which grows in the high Andean plains of Bolivia, Ecuador, Peru and Colombia.

The coca plant

The South American Indians who grow and harvest the

coca plant sometimes use it to ward off the effects of hunger. They are mostly poor people with little food to eat. They moisten a wad of leaf with saliva and give it flavor by the addition of crushed seashells or a cereal. Then they suck the wad between the gum and cheek. Some Indians chew a couple of ounces of leaves each day.

The leaves are particularly rich in vitamins and are thought to aid digestion. They may help breathing during hard work. (They are also supposed to help heal the strained voice box in the throat, which may explain the popularity of the old coca wines among singers and stage actors.)

Making cocaine

Much of the coca plant crop is illegal. But the harvest provides the South American farmers with a highly profitable crop they can sell to drug traders. The leaves are converted into a kind of paste in primitive laboratories and finally smuggled into better-equipped laboratories, mainly in Colombia, to be made into cocaine.

The leaves contain only one per cent cocaine. In the more sophisticated laboratories the paste is purified into the white cocaine powder.

The ritual of snorting

Cocaine powder or crystals are usually chopped or pressed into a finer powder, using the edge or flat side of a knife or

Cocaine in the making: liquid in the flasks of a "jungle laboratory."

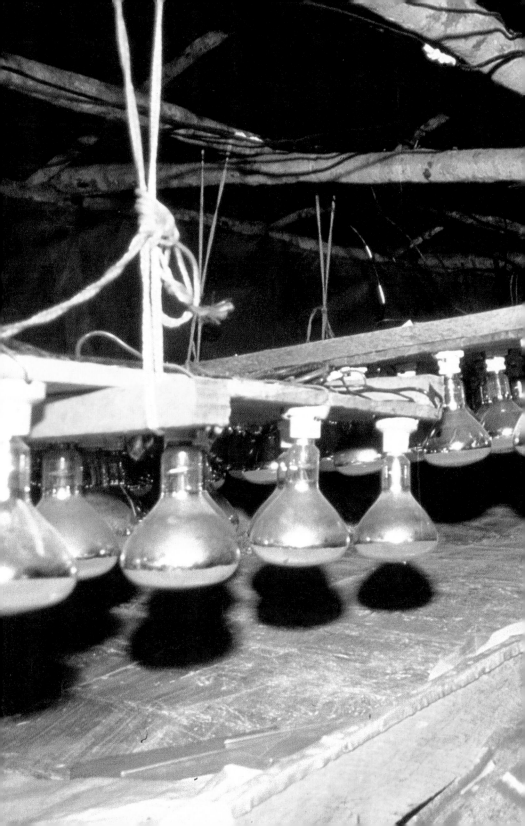

perhaps a razor blade. The powder is formed into short lines which are then sniffed hard, line by line, into one nostril at a time. This is called "snorting," one popular way of taking cocaine.

Any small tube can be used for snorting. Often it's something simple and cheap, like a straw. But the rich and famous have been known to use flashier implements like a rolled-up banknote or an expensively jeweled straw-shaped implement. This is because snorting can become something of an event, a ritual. But cocaine is water-soluble, which means it can be taken in other ways too. It can be taken orally, in liquid, and it can be smoked.

"Cutting" cocaine

Pure cocaine rarely reaches the streets these days. By the

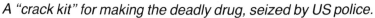

A "crack kit" for making the deadly drug, seized by US police.

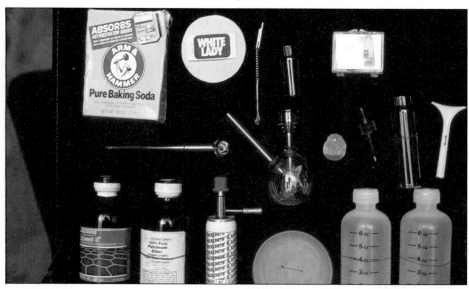

time it has gone through the chain of growers, refiners, smugglers, distributors and dealers, the powder has been bulked out or "cut" to make it go further. Drug traders add cheap substances like sugar, talcum powder or starch so it seems like they've got more cocaine to sell, and so they make bigger profits.

Heavy use and injecting

Some people prefer to inject their drugs and will try most things, including cocaine. For these people the bulking substances can be highly dangerous and even fatal.

There are also many serious risks from injecting, especially when needles or syringes are shared. These risks include hepatitis (a serious liver disease), blood poisoning (which can kill), and the deadly disease, AIDS.

Freebasing and speedballs

The process of "freebasing" is popular with some users. It involves smoking a form of the drug that has been treated chemically to separate out the "active" part of the drug molecule, which produces the effects. This is supposed to give a purer form of the drug that can be smoked ("ordinary" cocaine is not suitable for smoking).

The dissolved cocaine made by freebasing is usually smoked through a water pipe while the mixture is heated. Such pipes are available from many head shops. This way of taking cocaine is often the only way left for heavy users whose noses have become too damaged by prolonged snorting or whose veins have been destroyed by frequent

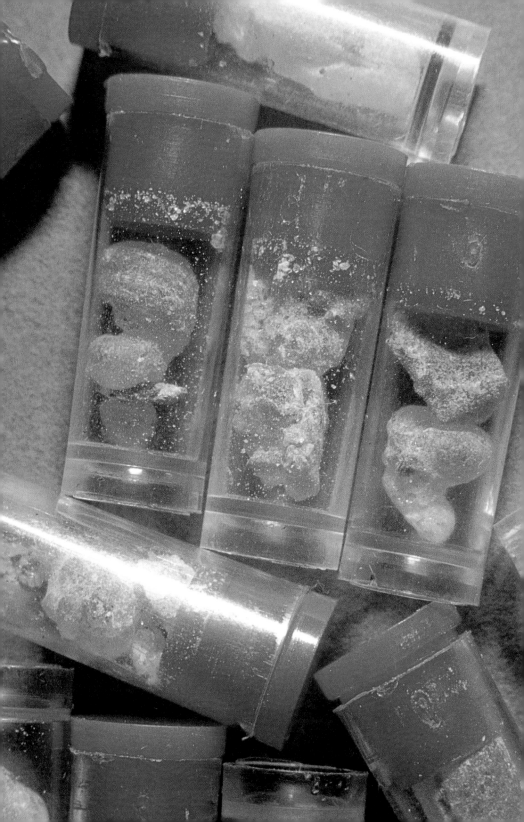

injections.

Another way of taking cocaine is in combination with heroin, the so-called "speedball." A deadlier combination is hard to imagine.

The "marketing" of crack

Why was crack "invented?" Some people say that snorting a drug up the nose was not quite as acceptable as smoking a drug, inhaling it into the lungs. Cigarettes get away with being smoked, yet they are deadly in their own way.

So the drug "barons" who grow and distribute drugs, and the traders who spread them into the local network, looked for a way of smoking cocaine. There was a lot of cocaine about, too, as the growers increased their crops to make more profits.

Eventually a way was found to change cocaine into a simpler form which could be smoked and was cheap. Crack had arrived. Its popularity is also due to its faster and more explosive effect than cocaine. In the language of the marketing world, it was a "good product." Which meant that more people would take it and more people would become ill and die as a result.

Making crack

Crack is made by mixing cocaine crystals with a few simple chemicals until the mixture becomes a paste. After cooking, the paste hardens into small pellets or rocks. The cooking

Death and misery in little bottles – crack rocks from a drugs bust.

gets rid of some of the unwanted chemicals from the cocaine, leaving a purer and more powerful substance.

The chips of rock are usually smoked on an improvised pipe, for instance a beer can with a few pinholes in it. The crack is burned with a match. As the rocks heat up and give off their smoke they tend to pop and crack, hence the name "crack."

The risks of crack

Crack has many unpleasant side-effects. In a survey of people who had been taking crack, two users out of three said they had chest and breathing problems. Two out of five had a continually bad cough. Almost nine out of ten were suffering from bad depression. Two out of five said their memory was worse and they forgot things.

One in three crack users behaved violently. And over half became paranoid, suspicious of everyone around them.

Perhaps the most frightening result of the survey was that about one crack user in five had attempted suicide. This was partly as a result of all the other effects of the drug, such as depression and paranoia, ganging up together. In the end, killing yourself seemed the only escape (though of course this is not true).

Paranoia was a special problem. Some crack users believed that everyone, even those who were trying to help, were really out to trick them. They thought that people were talking behind their backs and laughing at them. This made admitting the problem, and seeking help, even more difficult.

ARE COCAINE AND CRACK ADDICTIVE?

"I just tried it once, to see what it was like."

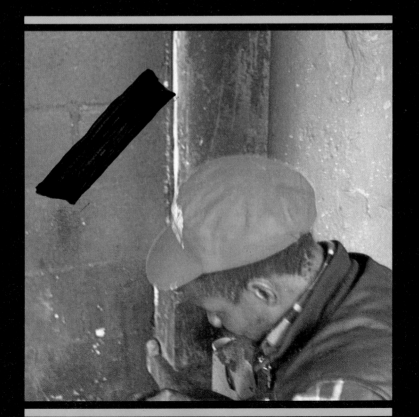

Cocaine can be an addictive drug. It's not quite the same as a drug like heroin, when the body comes to depend on regular doses and reacts violently if these are taken away. Addiction to cocaine is more a mental dependence, an addiction of the mind.

To many people the use of cocaine still means excitement, success and glamor. This is not true today – and in fact it never has been. One problem is that a lot of people are unaware of the dangers cocaine poses to their health. They see no reason to stop repeating what seems like a pleasurable sensation.

New users of cocaine

The stranglehold that cocaine has on the public is shown by the increasing numbers of people who have tried the drug at

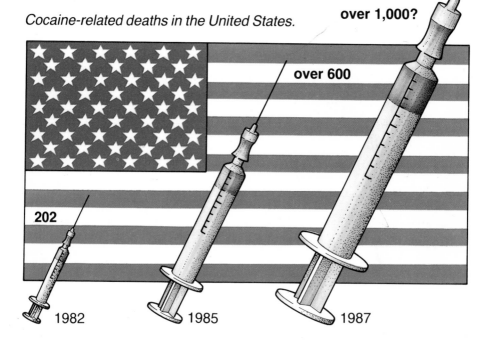

Cocaine-related deaths in the United States.

over 1,000?

over 600

202

1982   1985   1987

least once (the "ever-users"). These have gone up from five million to more than 20 million. It is estimated that there are around five million regular users of cocaine in the United States alone and that about 5,000 people a day try this drug for the first time.

Cocaine use is also increasing in Europe. The latest estimates show that the numbers are going up by one third each year in Italy and by one half each year in West Germany and Britain.

Regular cocaine use

The more regularly someone uses cocaine, the less effect it begins to have. The brain gradually gets used to the drug. This is called tolerance. Higher and higher doses are needed to get back the stimulating effects, so more and more cocaine is needed, and the costs and risks go up.

There is no greater imprisonment than that of being dependent on any chemical substance for one's existence.
(Stacy Keach, American actor and convicted cocaine smuggler.)

Crack: instant addiction

Some people claim that cocaine is not very addictive or that they can easily control its use. But there seems little doubt that crack is extremely addictive.

Simple and natural curiosity, to find out for yourself what all the fuss is about, is one common reason for trying crack. At only a few dollars for a "hit," most people can afford this one time experience. Some drug pushers actually give crack away for free to first-timers. They know that some of the users will become addicted and become regular customers, and their profits will therefore increase.

❝❝ I just tried it once, to see what it was like. ❞❞

What if the first-time users knew what the experts estimate? That as many as three out of every four first-time crack users become instantly addicted? This makes their chances of not becoming an addict as low as one in four. Would they try it then, "just to see?"

Part of the problem, again, is that smoking crack somehow does not have such a bad image. "Snorting," when taking cocaine, is for some reason worse. This view has led many people to believe they will not become addicted to crack. But the facts are against them. The intensity of the addiction can be terrifying and horrific.

❝❝ A 16-year-old boy hacked his mother to death because she tried to stop him taking crack. ❞❞

Paying for crack addiction

Some people who take crack have to steal continuously, or get involved in some other crime, to pay for their addiction.

In young people it usually starts with theft from parents or relatives. But the addiction can become so strong that young people will take enormous risks to steal, from homes

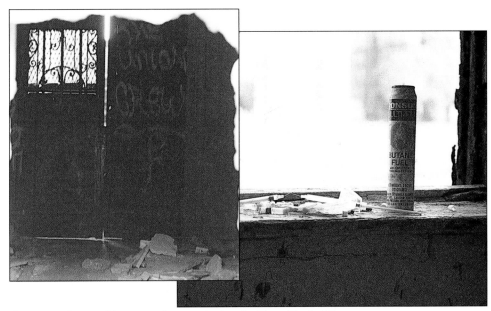

The squalor and horror of a crack den in New York City.

or shops or wherever, so that they can raise the money to buy crack.

With adults, bank balances suffer first. Then they borrow from friends, sell the car and hi-fi, and so on. A taxi driver sold his house to pay for his addiction and then hanged himself. A doctor's wife sold their baby for a few hundred dollars just to buy some crack.

Others take to prostitution, selling themselves for money or even for a couple of rocks of the drug itself. Some become dealers in crack itself, trying to make enough money to survive and to buy the crack they need.

The vicious circle

Within a couple of weeks of their first try, users may be smoking crack five or six times a day. They enter a vicious circle where the more they take, the more unpleasant the "crash" afterwards, and so the more they need to get high again. They are now addicted, taking crack not to feel good, but to stop feeling bad. They need crack to survive.

The crack explosion

The rapid rise in addiction to crack is like no other drug before. In one year the juvenile crime rate in Philadelphia doubled – almost totally as a result of youngsters needing money to pay for their crack addiction. It is estimated that one million people are using crack in the United States. The market has yet to explode in Europe, but the big-time drug dealers are trying to open it up and make even greater profits.

> ❝ If the Russians had wanted to find a way of destroying the youth of America, then crack would have been the perfect way of doing it. ❞

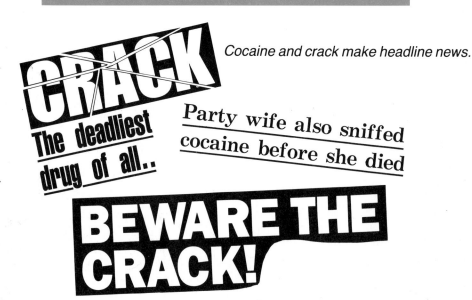

Cocaine and crack make headline news.

THE COCAINE AND CRACK TRADE

❝If I didn't carry the parcels, they would threaten my family.❞

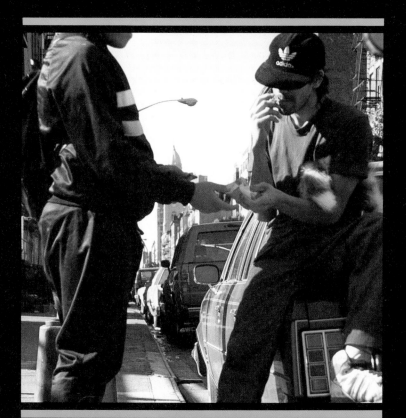

Selling crack and cocaine is a billion-dollar business. The drug barons are prepared to go to great lengths to protect such a high profit earner. Their products can cause misery and grief to millions of addicts. Yet the money generated by the coca trade is very important to the economies of several South American countries, even though it is mostly illegal.

For example, the export of cocaine is worth more than an estimated $1.5 billion a year to Peru, equivalent to about half the country's legal exports! Similarly, without the sale of cocaine, Bolivia's economy would be in much greater trouble than it is.

Bolivia and Peru together account for more than 90 per cent of the world's coca crop. In the past they have turned their raw coca paste over to the Colombians, who have exported it in the form of cocaine. Colombia is thought to produce more than three-quarters of the world's cocaine, with $5 billion from its sale coming into the country each year.

Coca in Bolivia

Coca plantations have sprung up all over Bolivia, from the high Andean slopes to the tropical plains in the Amazonian basin. More than a quarter of a million acres of coca plant are believed to be under cultivation. Of this, around four-fifths is destined for the illegal cocaine trade, with the other fifth being used in the legitimate drug industry and as food for the Indian population.

The country has no other way at present of creating enough wealth to offer an alternative to its people, especially since the world trade in tin collapsed. Workers have had to move to the coca-growing areas to earn money, to feed themselves and their families.

Coca – an obliging crop

Another reason why growing the coca leaf is so productive is that it is an ideal "cash crop." The plants mature in six months and the leaves can be picked six times a year. Compare this to bananas or oranges, where the trees can take up to three years to bear fruit.

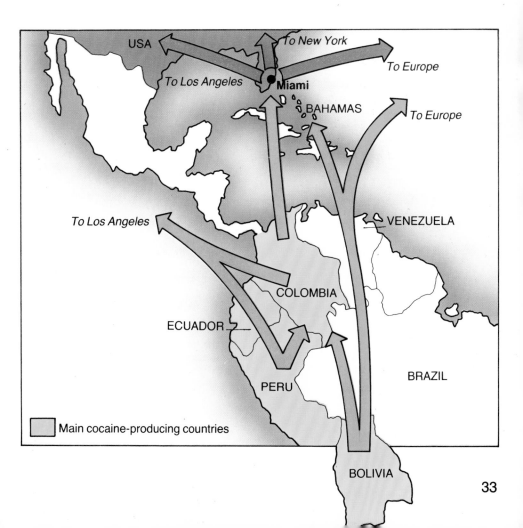

USA

To New York

To Los Angeles

To Europe

Miami

BAHAMAS

To Europe

To Los Angeles

VENEZUELA

COLOMBIA

ECUADOR

PERU

BRAZIL

Main cocaine-producing countries

BOLIVIA

In addition, the coca plant thrives when protected from the sun, in slight shade. So it can be planted beside taller crops such as corn, which hide it from officials hunting illegal crops.

In the past, South American countries have had little problem with cocaine abuse, compared to the United States and Europe. The wads of leaves that the Indians chew contain very little drug. Recently, however, cocaine addiction has begun to make an impact in South America. This is particularly in the form known as "bazuco," which is a stage in the processing of the coca leaf into paste, before it is turned into cocaine itself. Bazuco contains many unpleasant impurities not found in cocaine or crack. It is usually smoked in a cigarette, and addicts may smoke 30 or 40 of these cigarettes in a single session.

The big-time dealers

The sales of cocaine and crack are worth around $35 billion to South America. The coca plantations provide thousands of jobs for farmers. The amount of money generated by the cocaine trade runs to billions of dollars, but only a fraction returns to the countries which grow coca and make cocaine.

The rest is taken as profit by dealers, couriers and, of course, the drug barons who stash their money in foreign bank accounts. The illegal earnings are sent abroad and are "laundered" in the world financial markets, where it is easy to hide big transactions.

Coca leaves are harvested for processing into cocaine paste.

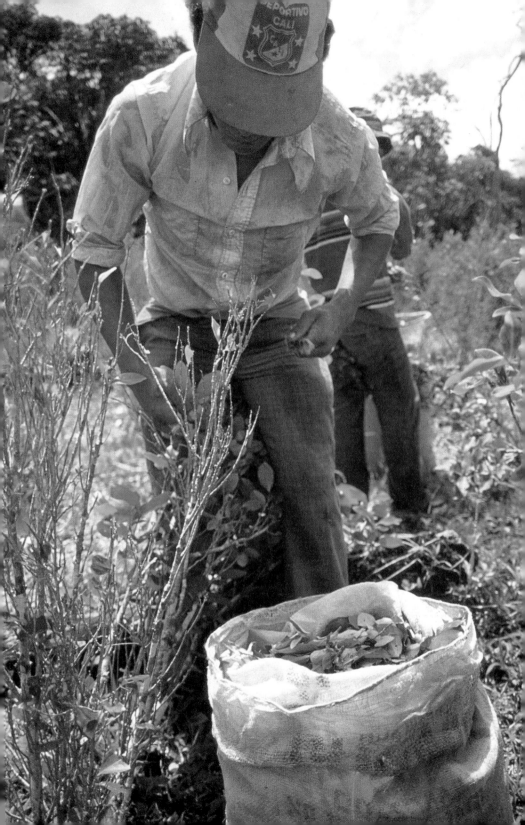

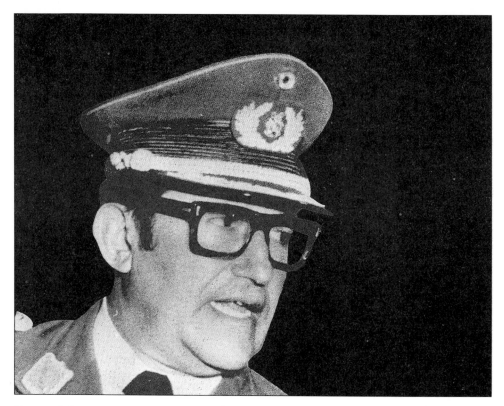

General Garcia Meza, heavily implicated in the cocaine trade.

A popular method of bringing money back into the country undetected is to buy high-priced consumer goods such as cars, aircraft and electronic equipment from overseas. The goods are smuggled into the country and sold on the black market for local currency.

Cocaine corruption in high places

Without their profitable coca crops, many South Americans would starve. So it is no wonder that some of their governments have not tried too hard to crush the cocaine business.

General Garcia Meza, formerly the president of Bolivia, was deeply involved in the cocaine trade. He even overthrew the Bolivian government in 1980, thanks to the support and money of the country's cocaine barons.

Because so much money is involved, murder and corruption have become a way of life to those in the cocaine trade. The Colombian drug barons were powerful enough to murder Chief Justice Minister Rodrigo Lara Bonilla in 1984. The barons are often able to escape because of the huge protective web they weave around themselves. Judges, customs officials and police officers are often in their pay.

The barons further protect themselves by getting others to take the risks and do their dirty work for them. In this way they can make millions without ever seeing or handling an ounce of cocaine themselves.

> ❝ **They controlled me completely. If I didn't carry the packages, they would threaten my family. They said they'd maim my baby.** ❞

Robbing the rich . . .

Despite their violent and corrupt lifestyle, many of the barons still regard themselves as "Robin Hood" figures. They believe that they rob from the rich (the cocaine users in wealthy North America and Europe) and help to feed the poor in their own country by buying their coca plants.

The drug barons may also try to make their images

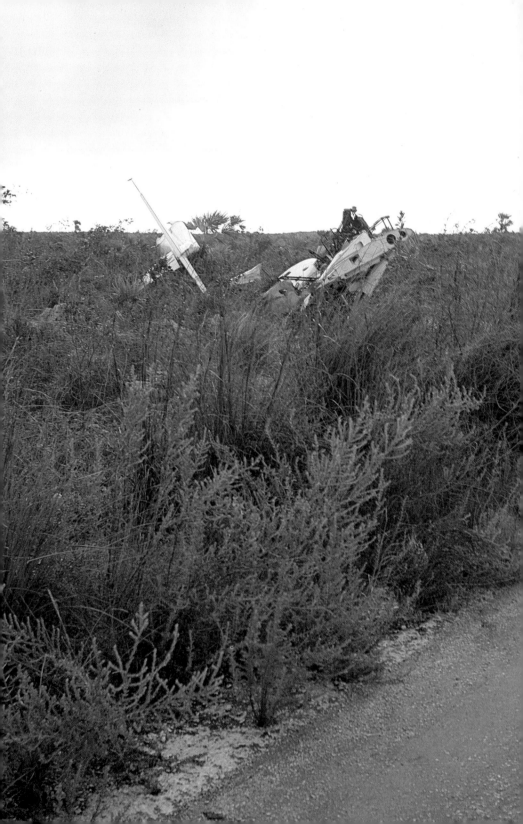

more respectable. They donate money to hospitals or schools, buy soccer clubs and put up money to buy star players, or even enter politics. Yet behind the scenes many of them are still involved in bribery, corruption and murder, letting nothing get in the way of their drugs empire.

Smuggling through the Bahamas

One of the most notorious drug barons of recent times is the Colombian Carlos Lehder, who smuggled millions of dollars worth of cocaine to Miami via the Bahamas. His smuggling was made easier after he bought one of the Bahama Islands, Norman's Cay. With the help of thugs and fierce dogs he terrorized the remaining people into leaving the island. He bribed Bahama police and officials to ignore the dozens of aircraft, loaded with cocaine, which landed on the island on the way to Miami.

Another smuggler who made use of the Bahamas was the Cuban-American Luis Garcia. He ferried drugs by plane via Rimini, the island nearest the US mainland. He is said to have paid off the police in a business that earned him millions of dollars.

In the same way that Lehder took over Norman's Cay, Garcia based himself on the island of Corda Cay. The local people had the choice of earning money from the cocaine racket or being tied up to trees while the smuggling went on. When the people Garcia was paying threatened him for a bigger slice of the profits, he turned them over to the Drug Enforcement Administration, in return for protection within the US legal system.

Crashed out on cocaine – a smuggler's light plane that didn't make it.

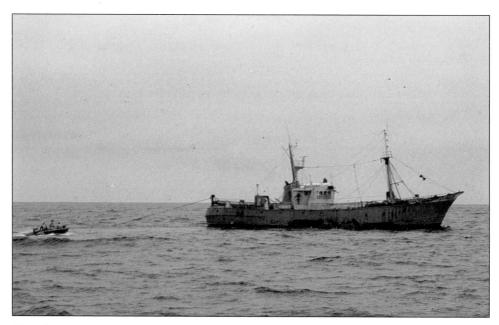

The Coast Guards approach a suspect ship on a search- and-seize mission.

Because the Bahamas have become the main stop-ping-off point for drug shipment between Colombia and the United States, many Bahamas people have themselves become addicts, with so much of the drug on their doorstep.

How the drugs are smuggled

The drug barons have become so powerful that it is common for them to have their own fleets of aircraft or speedboats, which they use to smuggle drugs from South America to countries in North America or Europe.

They are ruthless when it comes to their employees. A group of 40 Peruvians involved in the cocaine trade refused to obey orders, and they were massacred.

It is also easy to persuade very poor South Americans

to risk smuggling drugs on their person or in their luggage, though docks and airports. Small amounts of cocaine can make huge profits when sold on the street, so the couriers or "mules" do not need to carry much.

All kinds of ingenious methods of concealing drugs have been invented by the couriers. People have been known to swallow small plastic bags of cocaine, which are retrieved from the lavatory once they are through customs. They may pay with their lives using this technique. If one of the little bags breaks open the cocaine is absorbed into the body in a huge overdose which can kill.

Other smugglers hide the drug in the seams of their jeans, in children's toys, tubes of toothpaste or souvenirs. It has even been known for cocaine to be liquidized, sprayed on clothing, and then extracted by chemists from the material after the courier gets into the country.

Smuggling drugs in huge shipping containers is an easier way to transport them, since customs officials and coastguards rarely have the time to search a huge ship thoroughly.

Smuggling routes

Most of the cocaine which arrives in Europe is thought to come through Amsterdam, Madrid and London. Much of it is believed to come via Brazil, which has the most regular air services to Europe of any of the South American countries.

Colombia used to be the main exporter of cocaine to Europe, but over the last few years Bolivia has become what is thought to be the number one provider.

The cocaine trail ends on the street or in drug houses, as money and small bags change hands in the shadows.

Crack houses

The sale of crack has built up a culture of its own. "Crack houses" are places where crack addicts can go and smoke until their money runs out. These dens are common in run-down inner city areas in parts of New York and Miami. In New York alone there are thought to be several thousand crack houses.

Inside the house, the addicts are protected by armed drug dealers, huge steel doors and barred windows. Police have a tough time trying to catch the addicts and dealers, since by the time they have forced their way into the den, the crack (the evidence) has been flushed down the toilet.

Although crack is flooding the US market, it is still rare in Europe. But as the worldwide production of cocaine is greater than demand, it may be only a matter of time before the traffickers turn their attention to Europe.

THE BATTLE AGAINST THE DRUGS

❝*How can we find every little plastic bag?*❞

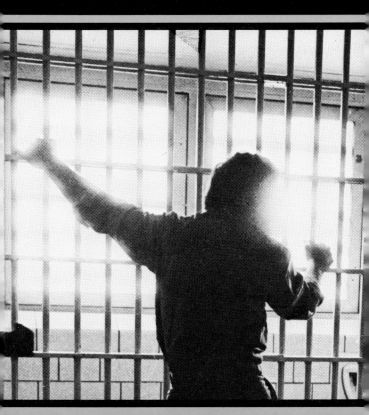

Western Governments have recognized the destructive influence of cocaine and crack on society. Once people are hooked on drugs, not only do their jobs suffer but so do their family and everyone associated with them.

This is why the US Government has decided to lead a strong attack against drugs. Thousands of millions of dollars have been spent on getting the message across: Cocaine is not a safe drug that anyone can control and crack is even more dangerous and can turn people into addicts overnight.

❝ It was a big delusion. I thought cocaine would make me all the things that I wanted to be – and it didn't work. ❞

The US government is trying not only to prevent the damage to people's lives but also to the economy as a whole. Drug abuse in the United States is estimated to cost industry more than $30,000 million a year in lost production, time off work and accidents.

Taking the fight to the suppliers

South American governments are keen to reduce the way their countries depend on drugs for money. Some can see the terrible situation of drug dealers gaining control over the entire economy. The governments of Bolivia, Peru,

Troops seize a cocaine shipment and throw it into the sea (inset).

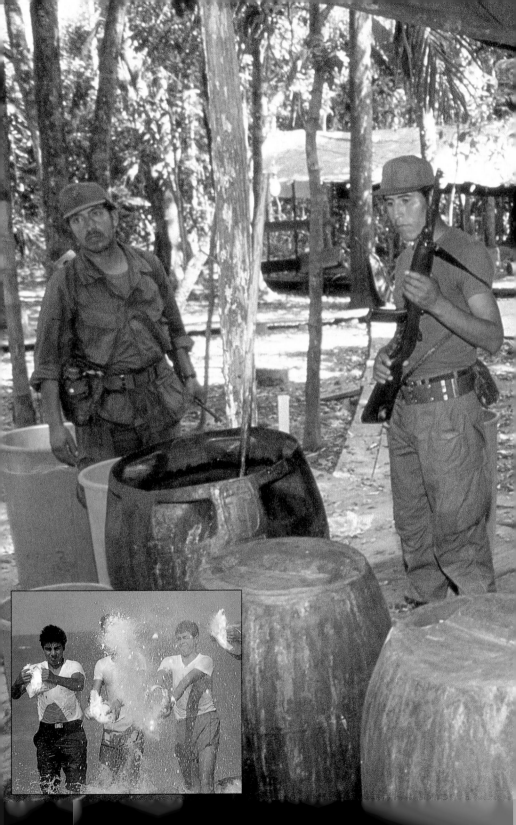

Ecuador, Colombia, and to a lesser extent Brazil, are beginning to fight the trade.

It is a dirty fight. The personal risks to those involved are high. Besides the killing of government officials, hundreds of Colombian police officers have been murdered or seriously injured in raids against traffickers who are heavily armed. Sometimes the traffickers have the support of anti-government guerrilla soldiers who take some of the drug profits in order to buy more weapons.

The battle in Bolivia

Bolivia showed it meant business when in 1986 US troops were sent to the country on the invitation of Bolivian President Victor Paz Estonoro. The president's action almost certainly resulted in the drug barons putting up a rumored $400,000 to have him killed.

During the raids, 160 US soldiers and six Black Hawk helicopters joined with the Bolivian army to deliver a blow to the cocaine trade. Illegal landing strips were blown up, jungle laboratories for purifying of cocaine were destroyed, and coca crops were burned.

This may have made only a small dent in the trade. But it did show that some South American governments wanted to assist the United States in their anti-drugs crusade. American agents and the Leopards, a special unit of the Bolivian national police, have meanwhile been seeking out and shutting down hundreds of paste laboratories in the Bolivian backwoods.

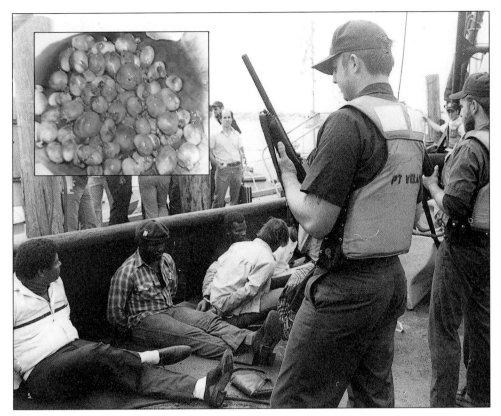

Suspected smugglers and (inset) drugs in a courier's stomach.

Colombia's crusade

When Colombian Justice Minister Lara Bonilla, who had spoken out against traffickers, was gunned down in the streets, the governments of South America came together. They feared a banding together of the drug dealers and anti-government guerillas.

Colombian officials agreed to an extradition treaty with the United States so that criminals could be caught in Colombia and then sent back to the United States for trial. They also allowed Drug Enforcement Administration agents into the country. Colombian forces have raided the southern

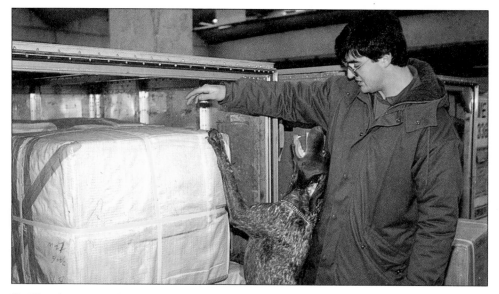

Sniffer dogs patrol docks and airports, trained to detect drugs.

jungle regions to wipe out cocaine-processing laboratories and airstrips.

The crusade had its ironical side. The local people had their livelihoods threatened, since many of them depended on the drug trade. At the same time some of them welcomed the raids, as they were paid by the drug barons to repair the runways.

Patrolling the borders

Attacking the source of cocaine is one of the many ways of fighting the battle against drugs. Patrolling the borders is another vital step in the fight although in the United States this is a difficult task with the borders thousands of miles long.

One major success against the cocaine smugglers was

in 1985 in Miami, the center of the illegal cocaine trade. Customs officers seized over a thousand kilograms of cocaine with a street value of $6 billion. The drugs were hidden inside flower boxes on a Colombian airliner.

The seizures of cocaine are increasing as officials become more watchful and more aware of the way drugs are smuggled across their borders. The United States government has recruited more officers and provided them with more sophisticated drug-detecting equipment.

Despite this, US police and customs officials estimate that they capture only about one-tenth of all drugs smuggled into the country. So despite extra efforts large amounts of cocaine and other illegal drugs are still finding their way across the borders and eventually onto the streets.

How can we cope? We can't even stop the wetbacks and all the other bods from coming over. How can we find every little plastic bag?

Cocaine in Europe

In Europe the amount of cocaine seized has increased by more than 12 times in the past 10 years. The British government expects that South American drug traders will try to smuggle even larger quantities into Europe in the next few years.

Aware of the potential problem, the British government established a Cocaine Target Team at Customs headquarters in London, in 1984. Its aim was to improve the "intelligence" coming back from informers and undercover agents, so that investigators now stand a better chance of catching cocaine smugglers and traders.

There have been successes already. Osvaldo and Magnus Bernardi, the sons of a Brazilian judge, were caught smuggling 13 kilograms of cocaine into London with a street value of $3.75 billion.

The British government is also trying to help South American countries fight the cocaine trade. Britain has given $900,000 to Bolivia to help its police force with training and equipment. In 1986 the government promised $1.5 million to help equip and train local police forces especially in the city areas, in the fight against cocaine.

Taking the war onto the streets

Once cocaine reaches the streets, local police and law enforcement agencies take over. Police forces all over the world are being strengthened to try and stem the flood of cocaine and crack abuse. For example, the New York police force recently created a 300-man anti-crack squad while London police increased their anti-drug squad by 50 to 200.

In the United States the risk of arrest does not seem strong enough to stop dealers selling drugs. Even if the dealers are caught, the prisons are so overcrowded already that they often spend only a few days locked up before they are out to await trial. Although there are more arrests, more convictions and longer sentences for drug offenses than ever before, this is a reflection of the increasing volume of drugs being sold rather than the fact that the police are winning their battle.

Prisons are often so overcrowded that they cannot take any new prisoners. Thus, drug traders may get off with lighter sentences than many people feel they should have.

Drug Tests for all?

Other measures to try and curb drug abuse have included compulsory drug testing by many United States companies. Workers have to give a sample of their urine for analysis which shows if they have been taking drugs. This has had some success in cutting down drug abuse.

The message is clear: crack destroys life.

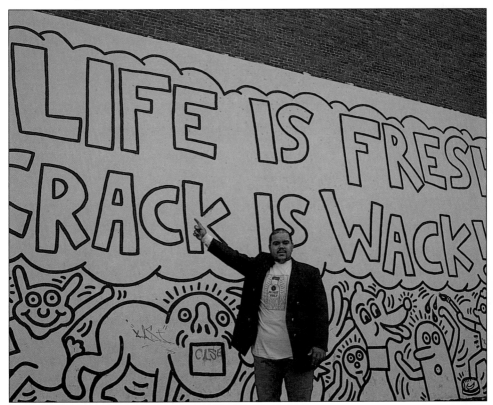

These tests have been very controversial. Some people say that they are an invasion of privacy. They say the tests mean that someone is assumed to be guilty of drug abuse until proved innocent – which goes against our traditions of common law and justice.

Advertising and publicity

Western governments have also taken to advertising campaigns to warn people of the dangers of drug abuse. Musicians, film stars and other celebrities have joined the anti-drugs campaign so that people who look up to them are discouraged from taking cocaine and crack. Benefit concerts and other events raise money to fight drug abuse. The bottom line for attacking the cocaine and crack problem is to let people know about the terrible effects that cocaine and crack can have on lives. Many experts say that this is the only way of really winning the battle. Some say that schools should have drug education classes, so that from an early age we can come to understand the dangers.

The "Just Say No" campaign has tried to persuade young people that they have the right to say "No." It is not being uncool or nerdlike to say no. It is being independent, confident and free.

"Just Say No."

GETTING HELP

" . . . a willingness to fight addiction is vital. "

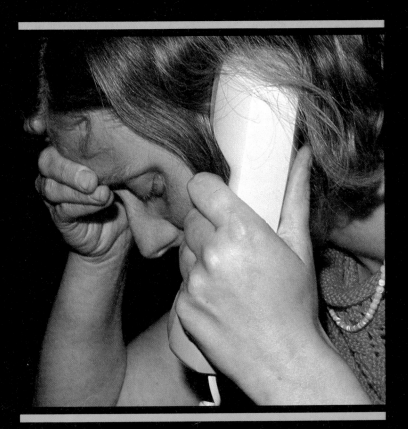

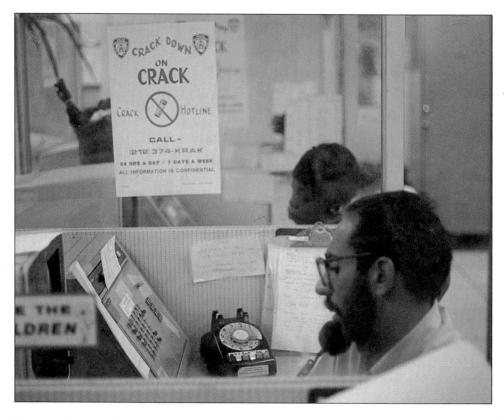

The crack explosion keeps the hotlines busy with people in trouble.

Addiction to crack or cocaine is not incurable. Many countries have set up drug centers to help drug users beat their problem. There are also many private organizations that get money from charities and fund-raising events.

The early stages

The most important part of beating drugs is for the user to say, honestly, that he or she wants to give it up. Other people can help, talk, give counsel and advice. But in the end it is up to users who must promise themselves that for advice and help.

Users are helped to come to terms with a drug-free life. They are given advice so that they can find for themselves new ways of spending their time, using their skills, and coping with the problems of life. This is called rehabilitation, or rehab. It often means breaking with the old routine and seeing less of associates who are still involved with drugs.

Private and state clinics

There are private drug clinics in most North American and European countries. They provide expert care, but many who need help cannot afford to go there, either because they come from a poor background or because their habit has eaten away their savings and jobs.

In most cases of drug abuse it's understanding, not punishment, that will help to find the solution. But a willingness to fight addiction is vital. So is an understanding of the problems and damage which drugs can cause. However, it is a battle that many users and addicts have won, returning to a drug-free normal lifestyle.

The striking symbol of the anti-crack campaign: crack down on crack.

FACT FILE

What cocaine and crack look like

Cocaine is made from the leaves of the coca plant, scientific name *Erythroxylon coca*. This is a leafy shrub that grows 6 to 8 feet tall. (It is different from the cacao tree, from which come chocolate and cocoa "drinking chocolate.") Coca plants are grown mainly in warmer parts of South America, where they originally come from, and also in Africa, Southeast Asia and Australia.

To make cocaine, the leaves are processed in a laboratory into a paste,

Pure cocaine powder.

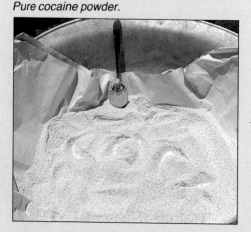

which is then changed by another chemical process into a white crystalline powder, cocaine hydrochloride. This is the drug cocaine, or "coke," sold illegally on the streets. By the time it reaches users it has usually been bulked out with sugar or similar substances. It is often called "snow," "sleigh-ride" or "white lady" because of its sparkling appearance.

Crack is made by heating cocaine with certain chemicals, so that it forms small light-colored pellets or "rocks." As these rocks are heated in order to breathe in the vapors, they pop and crackle, hence the name "crack."

Medically, cocaine was used as a local anesthetic to numb the surface of the eye or the inside of the nose or throat. (It was first used medically in 1884 by Carl Koller, an eye surgeon.) It is rarely used in medicine now.

Tell-tale signs of drug abuse

If you suspect someone of secretly taking drugs such as cocaine and crack, there are several tell-tale signs which include:

- sudden bursts of energy, not wanting to eat, pupils of the eyes dilated (widened) giving a staring look
- equipment used to snort cocaine such as a mirror (to arrange the powder on), a razor blade or knife for crushing the powder and arranging it into "lines," a straw or tube for sniffing, perhaps with a Y-shaped end for sniffing into both nostrils at once
- a pipe-like item such as a beer can with holes punched in it, for heating crack and inhaling the fumes, and boxes of matches or lighters hidden away

Emergency

If someone gets into trouble with drugs, such as becoming unconscious, summon immediate medical help. While waiting, place the person in the recovery position, shown below. This way, if he is sick, he is less likely to choke on the vomit.

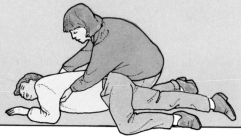

DRUG PROFILE

Common name	Cocaine
Other names	Coke, snow, lady, charlie
Drug name	Cocaine hydrochloride
Drug type	Stimulant
Made from	Leaves of the coca plant, dried and processed chemically into a paste and then into a sparkling powder
Ways of taking	Mostly by sniffing through a tube up the nose ("snorting"); some users inject
Main effects	Increased alertness and feelings of energy; lack of tiredness; followed by feelings of worry and fear, possibly hallucinations; larger doses may cause inability to sleep, trembling and fits, breathing problems, skin sensitivity and digestive trouble
Addictiveness	Often psychologically addictive; physical addiction is more debatable
Other effects	Dilated pupils; loss of appetite; increased heart rate and blood pressure; dry lips; sores and ulcers in the nose from too much snorting; ulcers and abscesses on the skin at injection sites
Withdrawal effects	Mainly psychological and include hunger, tiredness, depression and worry, apathy, irritability, disorientation

Common name	Crack
Drug type	As for cocaine
Made from	Chemically processed from cocaine or the paste from which cocaine is purified
Ways of taking	Smoking, by heating the drug and inhaling deeply into the lungs
Main effects	As for cocaine but faster, more intense and powerful
Addictiveness	Still a relatively new drug but studies show severe addictiveness, with people becoming "hooked" after only one session
Main producer countries	Coca leaves for cocaine and crack come from several South American countries, especially Peru, Bolivia, Colombia, Ecuador
Main consumer countries	Most countries of the Western world, with numbers of cocaine users going up rapidly; an estimated one million regular cocaine users in the United States
Example of cost	$80 to $125 for a gram
Legal status	Under the Controlled Substances Act, the sale or possession of cocaine (including crack) is illegal
Penalties	Sentencing varies from state to state, but Federal Law imposes severe penalties for being involved with cocaine or crack

SOURCES OF HELP

Here are addresses and telephone numbers of organizations that might be able to help people with a drug problem.

National hotlines
National Cocaine Hotline
1 (800) C-O-C-A-I-N-E
This is a national toll-free number that provides callers with counseling twenty-four hours a day.
National Institute on Drug Abuse -
Treatment Referral
1 (800) 622-H-E-L-P
This hotline is staffed from 9.00am to 3.00am on weekdays and from 12 noon to 3.00am on weekends. Counselors can talk with you, refer you to a drug treatment program, or answer questions about drugs, treatment, health or legal problems.
New York State Division of Substance
Abuse
1 (800) 522 5353
This toll-free number reaches counselors who can provide referrals for treatment or legal advice, or over-the-telephone crisis intervention.
National Federation of Parents for Drug
Free Youth
1 (800) 554-K-I-D-S
This is not a crisis hotline, but a place to call for drug information. This educational organization provides both parents and kids with informational pamphlets, books, and videos.

Self-Help Organizations
Cocaine Anonymous
263A W 19th Street
New York, NY 10011
(212) 496 4266
This is a self-help group modeled on Alcoholics Anonymous. To find a local chapter near you, call the number above.
National Self Help Clearinghouse
33 W 42nd Street
New York, NY 10036
(212) 840 1259
Can provide information on self-help rehabilitation organizations in your area, or put you in touch with one of the twenty-seven state and local self-help clearinghouses around the country.

Drug Treatment and Rehabilitation Programs
There are 8,000 to 10,000 drug treatment programs across the country. These include inpatient (residential) and outpatient facilities, covering a range of services: detoxification, counseling, family intervention, aftercare. Call one of the national hotlines to find a program near you. Also, your local hospital may be able to direct you to a treatment program. Or check the Yellow Pages under Drug Abuse and Addiction.

Referrals, information and more
Hale House for Infants
68 Edgecombe Avenue
New York, NY 10031
(212) 690 5623
This Harlem, New York, center takes care of the children of drug addicts.
Freedom from Chemical Dependency
26 Cross Street
Needham, Mass. 02194
Besides conducting drug prevention workshops in schools for faculty and students, this organization offers "evaluations" – after two meetings, a counselor can refer the client to an appropriate drug program. Also provides family intervention.
National Association on Drug Abuse
Problems
355 Lexington Avenue
New York, NY 10017
(212) 986 1170
Conducts a drug prevention program and offers family counseling.

WHAT THE WORDS MEAN

addict someone who needs to keep taking a drug in order to remain "normal" and stave off withdrawal effects on the body and/or mind. "Addiction" has a slightly different meaning to "dependence," in that it usually refers to someone who has been dependent on a drug for some time, and it is more tied up with his or her lifestyle and society's view of him or her.

cocaine a stimulant drug made from the leaves of the coca plant

crack a stimulant drug, a purer and chemically "base" form of cocaine which can be smoked

dependence the need to keep taking a drug regularly, either for its effects on the body (to keep away withdrawal symptoms, for instance) or its effects on the mind (such as to make the user think he is "getting through the day"). Dependence caused by cocaine and crack is largely psychological

drug any chemical or other substance that changes the body's workings (including the way the person's mind works, his or her behavior, etc.)

drug abuse non-medical drug use with harmful effects on the abuser and possibly on others

drug misuse using drugs in a way which people in general would see as not sensible, or not acceptable, and possibly harmful

snorting sniffing a drug up into the nose, usually applied to cocaine

stimulant a drug that stimulates the body's nervous system, especially the brain, to give feelings of increased alertness, physical and mental strength and energy. A stimulant also tends to banish feelings of tiredness, hunger and pain. Many mild everyday drugs, such as the caffeine in tea and coffee, are weak stimulants

tolerance when the body becomes used to a drug, so that the same dose begins to have less effect, and increasing doses must be taken for the same effect. In general cocaine use does not lead to tolerance, but this is more likely with crack

upper drug slang for a stimulant, sometimes applied to cocaine but more often to amphetamines ("speed" or "pep pills")

withdrawal the effects on the body and mind when a person suddenly stops taking a drug after being dependent on it. The effects are usually unpleasant and with cocaine may include depression, tiredness, apathy and hunger

INDEX

Photographic Credits:
Cover and pages 7, 25, 27 (both), 31, 51, 53, 54 and 55: David Browne; pages 4 and 22: John Hillelson Agency; pages 15 and 58: Hutchison Library; pages 19, 20, 35, 38, 40, 44 and inset, 47 and 48: Frank Spooner Agency; page 30: John Frost; page 36: Popperfoto; page 43: Newsday.

616.86 Chomet, Julian   c.1

Chomet   Understanding
             drugs: cocaine
             and crack

$11.90   -